Copyright © 2022 by Martina Giokos, RDN

Table of Contents

When shopping at the grocery store, the foods you grab can greatly impact your overall health. In fact, filling your cart with a lot of refined grains, sugary drinks, and processed foods can increase inflammation and affect your health.

Therefore, filling up on healthy foods can help keep you healthy, protect against chronic diseases resistant to drugs and rid your body of toxins.

We also absorb tons of toxins every day through the air we breathe, the water we drink, the food we eat, and by just being outside in our surroundings.

So how do we get rid of these toxins that can be harmful to our body? It's through the Healing diet.

The Healing foods diet is not just a diet; It is a tool that will lead you to a total transformation of your health. This diet was designed to help everyone overcome diseases. It is designed to heal your body and improve your health by encouraging the consumption of nutritious, whole foods like fruits, veggies, legumes, healthy fats, organic meats, and healing herbs and spices.

Plus, this simple eating pattern is a great way to ensure you supply your body with a steady stream of the nutrients you need to help prevent nutritional deficiencies in your diet and to promote healthy living.

So what makes this diet unique?

This diet is unique because it involves making some simple switches in your diet compared to other complicated diets with many rules and regulations.

1. Egg Roll in a Bowl (with chicken)

Prep: 10 mins

Cook: 10 mins

Total: 20 mins

Servings: 2

Ingredients

- 2 1/2 cups cabbage, chopped
- 2/3 cup carrots, grated
- 8 oz chicken breast (ground or chopped)
- 1 tbsp tamari sauce
- 1 cup cauliflower, chopped
- 2 tbsp olive oil
- 3 tbsp toasted sesame seeds
- 3 garlic cloves, minced
- 2 scallions, chopped
- Optional: turmeric and crushed red pepper flakes

Directions

1. Chop all vegetables and the chicken (if not ground).

2. In a large pan, heat some olive oil (or coconut oil) at medium-high heat saute the 2 cloves of garlic for 30 seconds, then add the chicken and the cauliflower. Saute everything for 4-5 minutes (until the chicken is almost ready)

3. Add in the cabbage, carrots and stir in the tamari sauce and the other garlic clove. Cover with a lid and cook for 4-5 more minutes or until the chicken is done. Optionally you can also add some turmeric and crushed red pepper flakes.

4. Serve with toasted sesame seeds and scallions.

Prep: 30 mins

Cook: 10 mins

Total: 40 mins

Servings: 4

Ingredients

- 2/3 cup low-sodium soy sauce
- 2 tbsp honey
- 2 tsp sesame oil
- 2 cloves garlic, minced
- 2 tsp grated fresh ginger
- 1/4 tsp crushed red pepper flakes
- 1 1/2 Ibs skirt steak, cut into 1-inch thin slices
- 1 tsp canola oil
- 2 1/2 cups broccoli florets

Directions

1. Whisk soy sauce, honey, sesame oil, garlic, ginger, and red pepper flakes in a bowl. Place steak in a shallow dish. Pour half the marinade over steak. Marinate for 20 minutes. Save leftover marinade.

2. Heat the canola oil in a large nonstick skillet or wok over high heat. Remove beef from marinade and cook 5 minutes.

3. Add broccoli and remaining marinade and stir-fry up to 5 minutes, or until broccoli is crisp-tender. Serve beef mixture over rice, if desired.

Prep: 8 mins

Cook: 12 mins

Total: 20 mins

Servings: 3

Ingredients

- 10oz/ 280g chicken breast, cut in strips
- 1 ½ tbsp olive oil
- 3 garlic cloves, minced
- 2 cups zucchini, chopped
- 1 bell pepper, chopped
- 1 cup frozen peas
- 2 cups rice, cooked
- 1 ½ tbsp tamari sauce
- 3 scallions, thinly chopped

Directions

1. Cook the chicken with olive oil for about 4 minutes. Then add the zucchini, garlic and bell pepper. Saute for 2 minutes, then stir in the peas for 3 more minutes.
2. Add in the cooked rice and tamari sauce, letting the rice toast and stirring occasionally for the next 2-3 minutes.
3. Lastly, stir in the scallions and turn the heat off after about 1-2 minutes.
4. Enjoy!

4. Beef Sirloin Teriyaki

Prep: 30 mins

Cook: 10 mins

Total: 40 mins

Servings: 4

Ingredients

- 4 (Four) 6-oz Sirloin Steaks
- 1/3 cup of Low-Sodium Soy Sauce
- 3 tbsp of Brown Splenda
- 1 Garlic clove, minced
- 1 tbsp of Ginger
- 1/2 teaspoon Crushed Red Pepper
- 2 tbsp Rice Wine Vinegar
- Salt and Pepper

Directions

1. In a small saucepan, over medium heat, combine the soy sauce, brown splenda, vinegar, ginger, garlic and red pepper

2. Bring to a boil and cook 5 minutes

3. Remove from the heat and cool completely, about 15 minutes. Then, transfer the sauce in a large bowl

4. Add the steaks and let marinate for 30 minutes

5. Grill steaks until desired doneness

Prep: 5 mins

Cook: 40 mins

Total: 45 mins

Servings: 4

Ingredients

- 450g / 1 pound chicken drumsticks
- 500g / 1 pound sauerkraut
- 1 tbsp paprika
- 1 tsp crushed red pepper (optional)
- 1/2 cup bulgur, coarse
- 1/4 cup olive oil

Directions

1. Add all ingredients to a pot, add water or chicken stock, just enough to cover the ingredients, cover

the pot with a lid and cook at medium-high until boiling.

2. Reduce the heat and and let the meal cook for around 30 minutes or until the chicken and bulgur are done. During the last 5-10 minutes of cooking remove the lid. At any point after 10 minutes, add more water or stock if needed.

3. In the end, add salt and olive oil if needed.

4. Serve immediately - best with toasted bread! Store leftovers in an airtight container in the fridge.

Prep: 10 mins

Total: 10 mins

Servings: 1

Ingredients

- 1 tablespoon smooth natural peanut butter
- 1 ½ teaspoons sesame oil
- 1 ½ teaspoons rice vinegar
- 1 teaspoon maple syrup
- 1 teaspoon tamari or soy sauce
- 1 teaspoon water
- ½ teaspoon minced garlic
- Pinch of crushed red pepper (optional)
- 3 cups torn Boston or butter lettuce
- 3 ounces cooked shrimp
- ½ cup cooked brown rice
- ¼ cup chopped red cabbage
- ¼ cup julienned bell pepper
- ¼ cup julienned carrots

- ¼ cup julienned cucumber
- ¼ cup avocado
- Fresh mint and sesame seeds for garnish

Directions

1. Whisk peanut butter, oil, rice vinegar, maple syrup, tamari (or soy sauce), water, garlic and crushed red pepper (if using) in a small bowl until smooth.
2. Combine lettuce, shrimp, rice, cabbage, bell pepper, carrot, cucumber and avocado in a bowl. Add dressing and toss to combine. Garnish with mint and sesame seeds, if desired.

7. Creamy Keto Chicken and Vegetables

Prep: 5 mins

Cook: 15 mins

Total: 20 mins

Servings: 2

Ingredients

- 280g or 10 oz chicken thighs, skinless, boneless
- 3 scallions, thinly chopped
- 1 white button mushroom, roughly chopped
- 1 red pepper, chopped
- 1 tsp oregano, dried
- 2 cups broccoli, chopped
- 1 garlic clove, minced
- ½ cup Brussels sprouts
- ½ cup chicken broth
- 3 1/2 tbsp cream cheese
- 1/4 cup Parmesan cheese
- Salt and black pepper

- 1 tsp olive oil
- ½ cup mozzarella cheese

Directions

1. Wash the vegetables and the chicken. Chop chicken, broccoli and mushrooms, red pepper in bite-sized pieces, scallions thinly, Brussels sprouts in halves or quarters, and then mince the garlic.
2. Add the chicken to a pan with some olive oil, black pepper and oregano, cook at medium-high for about 5-6 minutes stirring occasionally.
3. Reduce heat to medium and move the chicken to one side of the pan, add the peppers to the other side. Allow the red pepper get fragrant for 1-2 minutes and then add in the broccoli, Brussels sprouts, mushrooms and scallions. Stir these in and cover the pan for about 3 minutes.
4. Add the chicken broth and minced garlic. Wait for about a minute or two for the broth to heat up, then stir in the cream cheese. Keep stirring until

all of the cream cheese has dissolved the sauce gets creamy.

5. Add the Parmesan cheese and stir until dissolved too.

6. Finally and optionally add the mozzarella cheese, salt and black pepper!

Prep: 5 mins

Cook: 30 mins

Total: 35 mins

Servings: 5

Ingredients

- 2/3 cup white rice
- 1 lb chicken breast, boneless, skinless
- 3 cups spinach, washed and chopped
- 1 cup canned chickpeas, rinsed and drained
- 1 carrot, shredded
- 6 scallions, chopped
- 2 garlic cloves
- salt and black pepper to taste
- 2 tbsp olive oil

Directions

1. Cook the chicken in the pan on both sides until golden brown.
2. Use the same pan and saute the onions and garlic for 30s with 1 tbsp olive oil.
3. At medium-high stir in the spinach, chickpeas, carrot and rice. Add salt and water to cover.
4. Cover with a lid and reduce the heat to medium. Cook until the rice is ready, stirring and adding water if needed.
5. Once the rice is done, add 1 tbsp olive oil and then salt to taste.
6. Add the cooked chicken and stir it in. Cook for 3-4 more minutes and add salt and black pepper if needed.

Prep: 2 mins

Cook: 8 mins

Total: 10 mins

Servings: 2

Ingredients

- 1/2 cup macaroni
- 1 1/2 cup cooked chicken, shredded
- 1/2 cup mozzarella
- 3 tomatoes, chopped
- 2 strings dill, chopped
- 2 garlic cloves
- 2 Tbsp olive oil
- 1 tsp tomato paste
- salt to taste

Directions

1. Remove the bones from the chicken thighs.

2. Place the chicken, chopped tomatoes, olive oil and minced garlic in a non-stick pan and cook at medium-high for 3-4 minutes until it starts looking like a tomato sauce.

3. Add a little bit of water (about 1/4 cup), some tomato paste, pinch some salt, stir in the macaroni and dill. The macaroni should be just covered, but not drowning in the sauce to cook properly.

4. Cook until the macaroni is ready, then stir in the mozzarella.

5. Let the mozzarella melt, making a cheesy tomato sauce.

6. Serve immediately!

Prep: 20 mins

Cook: 10 mins

Total: 30 mins

Servings: 4

Ingredients

- 1 1/2 lbs / 650g chicken breast, skinless, boneless
- 3 garlic cloves, minced
- 1 tsp chili flakes
- 1 tsp ground black pepper
- 1 1/2 tsp mint, dried
- 1/2 cup yogurt
- 1/2 tsp dill, dried or 1 tbsp fresh
- salt and pepper to taste

Hummus

- 1 cup chopped cabbage
- salad

- cooked broccoli
- 3-4 tortillas

Directions

1. Chop the vegetables for the salad and prepare the salad.
2. Make the garlicky yogurt sauce: mix the yogurt with 1 garlic clove, a pinch of salt and the dill until smooth.
3. Chop the chicken in bite-sized pieces and add it to a non-stick pan with 1 Tbsp olive oil, cooking at medium-high heat. Add 2 cloves of garlic, the chili flakes, black pepper and dried mint and stir together until the chicken is coated. Cook for 8-10 minutes or until the chicken is golden brown.
4. Assemble the wraps: Fill with as much as you like…In the center of a tortilla add the chopped lettuce or cabbage, the chicken, cooked broccoli (if using), some salad, the hummus and the tzatziki. Wrap like a burrito and enjoy immediately.

Prep: 5 mins

Cook: 30 mins

Total: 35 mins

Servings: 6

Ingredients

- 1 ½ Pounds Chicken Breast
- 2 Extra Large Egg Whites
- 1 tbsp Olive Oil
- ⅔ Cup Bread Crumbs - Whole Wheat
- 8 tbsp Parmesan Cheese - Grated
- ½ Cup Pasta Sauce
- ¾ Cup Mozzarella Cheese - Reduced Fat

Directions

1. Take out your Chicken Breast, trim the fat off of them, and cut them in half (so that they are thin)

2. In one smaller bowl add in your Egg Whites and
   Olive Oil

3. Mix those together

4. In another large bowl add in your Bread Crumbs
   and Parmesan Cheese

5. Mix those together

6. Take out a baking sheet, coat it with some non-
   stick cooking spray, and put your Chicken Breast
   onto your baking sheet

7. Lightly brush your wet mix onto both sides of
   your Chicken Breast slices

8. Dunk them into your dry mix

9. Coat the top of your Chicken Breast with some
   non-stick cooking spray

10. Put them into the oven on 450 degree F/232
    degree C for 20 minutes

11. Take them out, flip them over, and evenly
    distribute your Pasta Sauce + Mozzarella Cheese
    over the top of them

12. Put them back into the oven on 450 degree F/232
    degree C for another 5-10 minutes (or until your
    cheese is melted).

Prep: 5 mins

Cook: 15 mins

Total: 20 mins

Servings: 4

Ingredients

- 1 lb Ground Chicken (92/8)
- 1/2 Tbsp (8g) Chili Oil
- 1/2 C (96g) Swerve Brown Sugar
- 1/4 C (60g) Buffalo Sauce
- 2 tbsp (30g) Cider or Rice Vinegar
- 1 tsp Ground Ginger
- 1 tsp Garlic Powder
- 1/2 tsp Kosher Salt
- 1/2 tsp Black Pepper
- 1/2 tsp Red Pepper Flakes

Directions

1. Heat a skillet over medium-high heat with the chili oil. Brown both sides of the chicken, about 3-4 minutes per side, before mincing and fully cooking.
2. While the chicken cooks, whisk the remaining ingredients together in a mixing bowl.
3. Once the chicken is fully cooked, add the sauce to the pan and cook until thick and syrupy.
4. Serve with scallions and toasted sesame seeds over rice or cauliflower rice.

Prep: 15 mins

Cook: 20 mins

Total: 35 mins

Servings: 5

Ingredients

- 1 1/4lb raw chicken breast, chunks
- Crust
- 1/3 cup wheat flour
- 4 egg whites
- 1 1/2 cup (wheat) panko or wheat breadcrumbs

Orange sauce:

- 1 tablespoon coconut sugar
- 1 tablespoon soy sauce
- juice from 3 oranges (~3/4 cup)
- 1 tablespoon rice vinegar
- 1 tablespoon garlic, minced or paste

Optional For Added Flavor:

- 1 tablespoon of peanut oil or sesame oil
- 1 tablespoon ginger, paste
- 1 tablespoon (or more) Sriracha
- 2 teaspoons arrowroot starch + 1 tablespoon water

Note: Do Not Mix together until you add it to the skillet

Garnish:

- 1 tablespoon sesame seeds
- green onion

Meal Prep:

- 5 cups steamed broccoli (each meal has 1 cup broccoli)
- 2 1/2 cups brown rice or jasmine rice (each meal has 1/2 cup brown rice)
- low sodium soy sauce to taste

Directions

1. Set oven to 420 degrees F.

2. Chop chicken breasts into nugget-size chunks (or tenders if desired).

3. Beat the egg whites until somewhat frothy. Then toss the chicken in the whole wheat flour, then egg whites and then the panko crumbs. Place the coated nuggets on a baking sheet or baking rack. Bake in the oven for about 15 minutes until the outside is golden and crispy, and inside is white.

4. While it's baking, mix together the ingredients for the sauce except for the arrowroot starch.

5. Set a nonstick skillet on medium heat, then pour in the orange sauce. Bring it to a light simmer, then mix arrowroot starch with water and then pour it into the skillet. Stir immediately and quickly, then lower the heat and allow the sauce to thicken. Takes about 5 minutes.

6. Add the baked nuggets to a large bowl, then pour in the sauce. Toss the nuggets in the sauce and ensure they are all fully coated.

7. Garnish and enjoy immediately. If you're making this for meal prep, add about 1/2 cup of cooked brown rice (or jasmine rice) and at least 1 cup of steamed broccoli. Season to taste with low sodium soy sauce.

Prep: 20 mins

Cook: 14 mins

Total: 34 mins

Servings: 4

Ingredients

- 2/3 cup chickpeas, pureed
- 1/4 cup water
- 1/2 cup coconut flour
- 1/4 cup soy protein powder , vanilla or unflavored
- 2 tbsp granulated sweetener of choice
- 1/2 tsp baking powder
- 1/2 tsp baking soda
- 1/4 tsp salt
- 1 large egg
- 1/3 cup vanilla yogurt (Greek, Icelandic, non-dairy, etc)
- 1/4 cup milk of choice

- 1 tbsp coconut oil

- 1 tsp vanilla paste or extract

- 1/4 cup chocolate chips (milk, dark, non-dairy, etc)

Directions

1. Preheat the oven to 325 F. Grease a 12 cup muffin tin.
2. In a food processor or blender, puree the chickpeas with the water until smooth.
3. In a large bowl, add the coconut flour, protein powder, sweetener, baking powder and soda, and salt.
4. In a seperate bowl, combine the chickpea puree, egg, yogurt, milk, oil, and vanilla. Stir or whisk until fully combined.
5. Add the wet ingredients to the dry and stir until fully incorporated.
6. Fold in the chocolate chips.

7. Evenly distribute the batter into the prepared muffin tins. It will be about 1.5 - 2 Tbsps of dough per cookie.

8. Smooth out the batter so batter touches the edges of the pan, but don't press/flatten the dough.

9. Bake for 14 min. or until the edges of the cookies turn golden brown and a toothpick inserted into the center of the cookie dough comes out clean.

10. Allow the cookies to cool completely in the pan.

11. Feel free to top with nut butter, jam, or more chocolate.

Prep: 15 mins

Cook: 15 mins

Total: 30 mins

Servings: 1

Ingredients

Dough

- 1/2 cup self rising flour
- 1/4 cup fat free greek yogurt plain
- 1/4 teaspoon yeast this is for flavor only

Toppings

- 1/2 chicken sausage cooked
- 1/4 cup fat-free cheddar (kraft makes one)
- 3 tablespoon fat free feta
- 1/4 cup pizza sauce
- sliced onion, spinach, broccoli, mushrooms, or veggies of choice

Directions

1. Pre-heat oven to 475°C with a sheet pan in the oven. Make sure the rack is centered in the oven.

2. Mix flour, yeast, and greek yogurt together and stir until you get a shaggy dough. Work with your hands until you get a dough ball and there are no more bits of dry flour.

3. Shape dough into a ball and place in an oil (sprayed) square of parchment paper. Using another piece of oiled parchment paper on top, flatten and roll out using a rolling pin or bottle until it is about 1/4 thick. Remove top parchment paper. Total pizza size should be around 8" in diameter

4. Add toppings, transfer pizza to pre-heated sheet pan (leave on the parchment paper).

5. If you have a pizza paddle or another sheet pan, use that to transfer the pizza with parchment paper to the pre-heated pan. If not, you can remove the pre-heated sheet pan, transfer the pizza onto it, and then put it back in the oven. If

using another sheet pan, just use it upside down to transfer so the pizza can slide right off!

6. Turn oven down to 450°C and bake for 8 minutes. The top will be browning and bubbly.

Prep: 10 mins

Cook: 20 mins

Total: 30 mins

Servings: 4

Ingredients

- 1 pound boneless, skinless chicken breasts, trimmed
- ¼ teaspoon salt
- ¼ teaspoon ground pepper
- 1 7-ounce jar roasted red peppers, rinsed
- ¼ cup slivered almonds
- 4 tablespoons extra-virgin olive oil, divided
- 1 small clove garlic, crushed
- 1 teaspoon paprika
- ½ teaspoon ground cumin
- ¼ teaspoon crushed red pepper (Optional)
- 2 cups cooked quinoa

- ¼ cup pitted Kalamata olives, chopped
- ¼ cup finely chopped red onion
- 1 cup diced cucumber
- ¼ cup crumbled feta cheese
- 2 tablespoons finely chopped fresh parsley

Directions

1. Position a rack in upper third of oven; preheat broiler to high. Line a rimmed baking sheet with foil.

2. Sprinkle chicken with salt and pepper and place on the prepared baking sheet. Broil, turning once, until an instant-read thermometer inserted in the thickest part reads 165 degrees F, 14 to 18 minutes. Transfer the chicken to a clean cutting board and slice or shred.

3. Meanwhile, place peppers, almonds, 2 tablespoons oil, garlic, paprika, cumin and crushed red pepper (if using) in a mini food processor. Puree until fairly smooth.

4. Combine quinoa, olives, red onion and the remaining 2 tablespoons oil in a medium bowl.

5. To serve, divide the quinoa mixture among 4 bowls and top with equal amounts of cucumber, the chicken and the red pepper sauce. Sprinkle with feta and parsley.

Prep: 18 mins

Cook: 12 mins

Total: 30 mins

Servings: 4

Ingredients

- 5 tablespoons extra-virgin olive oil, divided
- 3 cups presliced fresh bell pepper-and-onion mix (10 ounces)
- 2 teaspoons white-wine vinegar plus 2 tablespoons, divided
- 1 pound shaved sandwich steak
- ¾ teaspoon ground pepper, divided, plus more to taste
- ¼ teaspoon salt, divided
- ½ cup shredded Gruyère or provolone cheese
- 8 cups baby arugula (5 ounces)

- 4 slices crusty whole-wheat bread (1/2 inch thick), lightly toasted
- 8 teaspoons prepared horseradish aioli or horseradish sauce

Directions

1. Heat 1 tablespoon of oil in a large skillet over medium-high heat. Add peppers and onions and cook, stirring often, until softened and starting to brown in spots, 5 to 7 minutes. Stir in 2 teaspoons vinegar. Transfer the vegetables to a bowl.
2. Add 1 tablespoon oil to the pan. Add steak, season with 1/2 teaspoon pepper and 1/8 teaspoon salt and cook, stirring and pulling apart with tongs or a fork, until no longer pink, 3 to 4 minutes. Return the vegetables to the pan, stir to combine. Sprinkle with cheese. Cover and remove from heat.
3. Toss arugula in a large bowl with the remaining 3 tablespoons oil, 2 tablespoons vinegar, 1/4 teaspoon pepper and 1/8 teaspoon salt.

4. Spread each piece of bread with 2 teaspoons aioli (or sauce) and top with one-fourth (about 1 cup) of the steak mixture. Serve the tartines with the arugula salad. Sprinkle with more pepper, if desired.

Prep: 5 mins

Cook: 10 mins

Total: 15 mins

Servings: 2

Ingredients

- 1 1/2 cup quinoa, cooked
- 1 1/2 cup shrimp, shelled and deveined
- 1 medium-sized tomato, chopped
- 1 cup spinach
- 1 cup zucchini, chopped
- 3 garlic cloves, minced
- 1 tsp crushed red pepper
- 1/3 cup mozzarella cheese
- 1 tbsp olive oil

Directions

1. Sear the shrimp on both sides for 2-3 minutes each side. Transfer onto a plate.

2. Use the same pan and add olive oil, the thinly chopped tomato, zucchini, garlic, spinach, some crushed red pepper and quinoa, cover and cook for 4-5 minutes until flavors combine.

3. Add mozzarella cheese melt, let it melt and then stir in the shrimp. Enjoy.

Prep: 15 mins

Cook: 10 mins

Total: 25 mins

Servings: 3

Ingredients

- 1 small head cauliflower or 2-3 cups cauliflower rice
- 2 tbsp tamari or soy sauce
- 2 tbsp olive oil or other oil
- 1 carrot, chopped
- 2 eggs
- 3 garlic cloves, minced
- 2 scallions, thinly chopped
- sesame oil (optional)

Directions

1. Grate the cauliflower or put it in your food processor to make your rice.

2. Chop the onion and carrot, mince garlic.

3. In a large non-stick skillet, heat 1 tbsp olive oil and lightly scramble the two eggs.

4. Once they're almost done, add the garlic and saute until fragrant.

5. Mix in your cauliflower rice, combine well. Let cook for about 2 minutes.

6. Add the other tbsp of olive oil and the tamari or soy sauce.

7. Cook for 3-4 minutes, stirring well, so that all the cauliflower gets covered with the tamari sauce.

8. Lastly, stir in the carrots and the scallions and cook for 2-3 more minutes. Add a tsp of toasted sesame oil (optional).

9. Serve hot and enjoy!

Prep: 15 mins

Cook: 20 mins

Total: 35 mins

Servings: 4

Ingredients

- 2 cups lentils (soak overnight)
- 1 carrot
- 6 broccoli florets
- 2 peppers (red or green, whatever you have)
- 1 fresh onion
- a handful of chopped cilantro
- 8 lime leaves
- 2 tbsp red curry paste
- 1/2 cup coconut milk/cream
- Optional: Serve with rice

Directions

1. Rinse the lentils after soaking overnight and put into a large cooking pan. Cover lentils with water and cook for 10 minutes at first at high and after 2 minutes at medium heat. If you're using small red lentils you might need less time.

2. In the meantime cut all the vegetables (carrot, broccoli, fresh onion, pepper) in stripes, chop cilantro.

3. When lentils are almost ready (you'll have to try them) - add 2 tbsp of the curry paste. Stir in well and add the coconut milk afterwards. Stir in well and leave to cook like that for 3-5 minutes, while stirring from time to time. Taste and add salt if you think you need it. If the lentils are not tender yet, add more water and cook while stirring a little longer. When ready continue to the next step.

4. Add lime leaves, cook for 1 minute and turn off heat.

5. Add all the vegetables and cilantro in the end. Stir in well, cover the pan with the lid and leave like that for a few minutes. Serve with rice if you want.

Prep: 5 mins

Cook: 5 mins

Total: 10 mins

Servings: 3

Ingredients

- 280g/ 10oz shredded chicken
- 2 tomatoes, chopped
- 3 garlic cloves, minced
- 1 cup arugula
- 3 tbsp chopped parsley
- 3 tbsp chopped basil
- 3 scallions, thinly chopped
- 1 bell pepper, chopped
- 1/2 cup canned chickpeas (optional)
- 1 tbsp olive oil
- 3 tbsp olives, chopped and pitted
- 1 1/2 tsp crushed red pepper

- 1 tsp coriander
- 1 tsp cumin
- tortillas

Directions

1. Boil and shred the chicken using two forks. While the chicken is boiling, toast the tortillas either in the oven or in a nonstick pan on the stove for 3-4 minutes until desired crispiness.
2. Wash tomatoes, bell pepper, scallions, and greens, then chop them. Peel and mince the garlic and prepare the spices to have ready to go.
3. Add the chopped tomatoes to a pan at medium-high, add in the rinsed and drained chickpeas, and start mashing these using a cooking spatula, cooking for about 1-2 minutes. (If you won't use the chickpeas and don't have fresh tomatoes, start with the next step).
4. Add in the shredded chicken, garlic, the crushed red pepper, coriander, cumin and olive oil (here's where you add tomato paste and a little bit of

water if you're not using the fresh tomatoes). In 1-2 minutes, stir in the peppers, olives and scallions. Keep stirring for another 1-2 minutes.

5. Last thing to do is stir in are the fresh herbs and greens (basil, parsley and arugula). Turn the heat off.

6. Top the toasted tortillas with this filling and fresh vegetables of choice like mashed avocado, tomato cucumber salad, more scallions, fresh basil or arugula.

Prep: 15 mins

Cook: 25 mins

Total: 40 mins

Servings: 3

Ingredients

Chicken

- 10oz/300g skinless boneless chicken thighs, in bite-sized pieces
- 2 tbsp paprika
- 1 tsp crushed red pepper flakes
- 2 tbsp dill
- 1 garlic, minced
- salt and pepper
- 1 tbsp olive oil

Cabbage salad:

- 2 cups cabbage

- 1 cup lettuce
- 2 tbsp dill
- 1 garlic clove
- 1 tsp vinegar
- salt and black pepper
- 2 tbsp chopped olives
- 1 tsp olive oil

Yogurt garlic sauce:

- 1/2 cup yogurt
- 2 garlic cloves, minced
- 3 tbsp dill
- salt

Additionally

- spicy roasted vegetables

Directions

1. Make the chicken. Mix chicken with the other ingredients in a bowl or directly in the pan, then cover the pan and cook for for 3-4 minutes at

medium-high. Take the lid off and stir for 6-7 more minutes or until the chicken is done.

2. For the salad add all ingredients to a bowl and mix them well together. (I recommend massaging the cabbage with vinegar or lemon juice and a little bit of salt first and then adding the rest of the ingredients).

3. Prepare the garlic sauce by mixing the ingredients in a small bowl.

4. Time to assemble your bowls: start with a base of the salad and then top with the chicken and roasted vegetables. Top everything with the sauce and enjoy!

Prep: 15 mins

Cook: 30 mins

Total: 45 mins

Servings: 3

Ingredients

- 2 tbsp. Coconut Oil
- 4 x 130g chicken breast
- 350g sweet potato
- 1/2 tsp. sea salt
- 1/2 tsp. black pepper
- 1/2 tsp. paprika
- 1 bag fresh spinach
- 350g green beans (trimmed)

Directions

- Preheat the oven to 180°C.

- Firstly, start by cutting your sweet potatoes into wedges and place onto a baking tray. Season with salt, pepper and paprika, then bake for 25 minutes.

- Boil the kettle and place the trimmed green beans in a bowl. Pour boiling water over the green beans with a pinch of salt and allow to blanch for 1-2 minutes (do not cook fully in order to retain nutrient value).

- Place the chicken breast on a griddle or large non-stick frying pan on a medium heat and cook until brown on one side, then flip the chicken over and flavour each breast with spices of choice

- Once chicken is thoroughly cooked place on a board to rest and cool.

- Drain the green beans from the salted water.

- Once all ingredients have cooled make up the the meal boxes. Add 2 handfuls of spinach, scoop of wedges, green beans and a chicken breast to each box.

- Store in an airtight container in the fridge, then microwave for 3-4 minutes or until piping hot.

Prep: 10 mins

Cook: 10 mins

Total: 20 mins

Servings: 3

Ingredients

For the pasta:

- 160g cooked pasta
- 3 breasts cooked chicken
- 2 stalks celery
- Handful cherry tomatoes
- 1 yellow pepper
- 2 tbsp. reduced-fat ranch dressing
- Large handful mixed leaves

For the buffalo sauce:

- 175ml peri-peri sauce
- ½ tsp. garlic powder

- 4 tbsp. reduced-fat butter or margarine
- Pinch salt

Directions

1. Place a saucepan over a medium heat and add the peri-peri sauce and garlic powder. Cook for 2 minutes, then add butter and salt and cook further for 5 minutes, stirring occasionally. Remove from the heat and allow it to cool for a few minutes.

2. Chop celery, tomatoes and pepper into bite-size pieces, and then shred the chicken using two forks. Place into a large mixing bowl with the cooked pasta.

3. Pour over buffalo sauce and toss it through the pasta salad. Divide amongst 3 meal-prep containers and drizzle a little ranch dressing over each, and serve with a handful of mixed leaves or your favorite side salad. Refrigerate for up to 3 days and enjoy hot or cold.

Prep: 15 mins

Cook: 35 mins

Total: 50 mins

Servings: 4

Ingredients

- 4 chicken legs (1.8 lb)
- 2 tbsp extra-virgin olive oil
- 1 onion, finely chopped
- 1/2 cup quinoa (washed)
- 1 cans chickpeas (1.5 cups chickpeas)
- 1.5 cups of hot water
- 1/4 cup dried cranberries
- 1 tsp ground cinnamon
- 1 tsp ground turmeric
- 1 tsp ground coriander
- 1/2 tsp crushed red pepper flakes
- 2 tsp salt

- 1 tsp black pepper
- 1 cup parsley (chopped)
- 9 oz cherry tomatoes (250g)

Directions

1. Season chicken legs with 1.5 tsp salt and 1tsp black pepper.
2. Now, heat the olive oil in the skillet, add the chicken legs skin side down and cook for 5 minutes. Then flip and fry for another 5 minutes until the chicken is nicely browned. Afterward, transfer the chicken to the plate.
3. Now, finely chop the onion and add it to the skillet. Right after that, add in cinnamon, turmeric, and coriander. Stir for 1 minute.
4. Add in washed quinoa and stir it so that spices coat it. Add 1.5 cups of hot water, give it a stir. Then, stir in the chickpeas and dried cranberries.
5. Add crushed red pepper flakes and the remaining 1/2 tsp of salt. Give it a stir.

6. Bring the chicken legs back into the skillet, bring the liquid to a boil. Then, reduce the heat and cover it with a lid.

7. Cook for 20-25 minutes until quinoa is tender and chicken is fully cooked. Let it sit for 5 minutes afterward.

8. Finally, divide the dish into 4 food containers. Chop some parsley and sprinkle it over each portion. Add in cherry tomatoes.

9. Refrigerate for up to 3-4 days.

Prep: 5 mins

Cook: 10 mins

Marinading time: 2 hrs

Total: 2 hrs 15 mins

Servings: 4

Ingredients

- 400 g turkey breast cut into chunks
- 2 tablespoon olive oil
- 2 pinch sea salt and black pepper
- 1 teaspoon paprika
- 0.5 teaspoon ground turmeric
- 0.5 teaspoon ground cumin
- 3 garlic cloves crushed
- 0.5 lemon juice only
- 5 g fresh parsley finely chopped

Directions

1. In a bowl, mix together the oil, spices, garlic, seasoning, lemon juice and parsley.
2. Put the turkey chunks into a bowl and add the marinade. Mix well and refrigerate for at least 2 hours.
3. Thread the marinated turkey onto pre-soaked skewers. Grill for 10 minutes, turning regularly.

Prep: 10 mins

Cook: 8 mins

Additional time: 2 hrs

Total: 2 hrs 18 mins

Servings: 4

Ingredients

- 3 lbs. Top Sirloin Steak diced into large 2 inch pieces
- 1/4 cup Fresh parsley chopped
- ½ Yellow onion quartered and pieces separated
- 2 cups Red Wine
- 2 tsp. Salt
- 2 tsp. Black Pepper
- 1 tsp. Aleppo Pepper optional

Directions

1. Begin by trimming and fat off the steak. Cut the steak into 2 inch size pieces across the grain.

2. Place the pieces into a mixing bowl. Season generously with salt, black pepper, and Aleppo pepper if using it. Add chopped parsley and the quartered onions.

3. Add the red wine and mix well. Cover with plastic wrap and allow it to marinade for at least an hour or two (longer if possible).

4. Preheat the broiler so it is set to high on your oven. Make sure the oven rack is as high as it can go with leaving room for the baking sheet to still fit.

5. Line a baking sheet with foil and place a roasting rack or cooling rack over the top to elevate the kabobs.

6. Cook for 3-4 minutes per side (this cooking time will vary depending on how rare you like your meat). Please note that every oven is different. You want the meat to sear but not get too dry.

7. Half way through, flip the kabobs to allow the other side to cook as well. Cook to 125-130 F. for medium rare. Continue to cook as needed if you prefer your steak with more doneness.

8. Remove from the oven and allow them to rest for 5 minutes. Remove the steak from the skewers and serve with your favorite sides.

Prep: 5 mins

Cook: 30 mins

Total: 35 mins

Servings: 4

Ingredients

- 2 cups brown rice, soaked
- 1 tbsp avocado oil
- ½ medium-sized red onion, chopped
- 1 red bell pepper, chopped
- 2 large carrot, peeled and chopped
- 5 cloves garlic, minced
- 3 1/3 cups low-sodium chicken broth or water
- ¼ cup liquid aminos
- 2 cups peas
- 1 pound boneless skinless chicken breasts, chopped into bite sizes

Directions

1. Soak the brown rice in water for at least 15 minutes (ideally several hours...up to 24). Drain the water completely and set aside.

2. Add the avocado oil to a large thick-bottomed pot and heat to medium-high. Add the onion, bell pepper, carrot, and garlic and saute for 3 minutes.

3. Add the rice and chicken broth, cover, and bring to a full boil. Reduce heat to a simmer and cook for 10 minutes. Add the chopped chicken and peas, stir well, replace the cover and cook for another 20 to 35 minutes or until the rice is tender and the chicken is cooked through.

4. Taste the rice for flavor and add sea salt and/or liquid aminos to taste.

5. Serve and enjoy!

Prep: 20 mins

Cook: 20 mins

Total: 40 mins

Servings: 4

Ingredients

- Pork
- 4 boneless pork chops (1-inch thick, ideally)
- 3 tbsp olive oil
- 1 tbsp honey
- 2 tsp paprika
- 1 teaspoon onion powder
- 1 tsp garlic powder
- 1 teaspoon dried oregano
- 1/2 tsp salt
- 1/4 tsp black pepper
- Vegetables
- 1 lb asparagus (trimmed)

- 1 red bell pepper (sliced)
- 1 green bell pepper (sliced)
- 1 yellow bell pepper (sliced)
- 2 tbsp olive oil
- 1/4 tsp of salt

Directions

1. Preheat the oven to 425 F. Begin by lining a baking sheet with foil or parchment paper.
2. In a separate bowl, combine olive oil, honey, paprika, onion powder, garlic, dried oregano, salt, and pepper.
3. Toss the pork in it, so it's fully covered with the mixture.
4. In a separate bowl, add in all the vegetables and toss in olive oil. Salt them and toss some more.
5. Spread the vegetables on the baking sheet but leave some space in the center. Place pork chops here.
6. Bake the pork with veggies in the oven for 15-20 minutes until pork chops reach 145 F

temperature. Try not to overcook the chops as they will dry out.

30. Banana Pecan Protein Muffins

Prep: 5 mins

Cook: 22 mins

Total: 27 mins

Servings: 12

Ingredients

- 3 medium ripe bananas
- 3 large eggs room temperature
- 2 tablespoon coconut oil melted and cooled
- 1 teaspoon vanilla extract
- 1 ¼ cup almond flour
- ½ cup vanilla protein powder
- ¼ cup ground flax seeds
- 1 teaspoon baking powder
- ¾ teaspoon cinnamon
- ½ teaspoon baking soda
- ¼ teaspoon salt

- 12 pecan halves plus about ¼ cup chopped pecans

Directions

1. Preheat oven to 350 degrees F. Grease a 12-cup muffin pan with oil or insert muffin liners. Set aside.

2. In a large mixing bowl, mash bananas until there are no large chunks left. Then add eggs, coconut oil, and vanilla, and whisk until well combined.

3. In a separate medium mixing bowl combine the almond flour, protein powder, flax, baking powder, baking soda, cinnamon, and salt. Add the dry mixture to the wet mixture all at once and stir with a wooden spoon or silicone spatula just until combined. Be careful not to over mix the batter.

4. Divide the batter between the prepared muffin cups, filling about ¾ full. Top each muffin with a pecan half and sprinkle with about 1 teaspoon chopped pecans. Bake for 22 to 28 minutes or until golden brown and a toothpick inserted

comes out clean. Remove the muffins from the oven and let cool for 20 minutes.